Breath Beyond Limits

A Compelling Guide to Conquer Cystic Fibrosis

Rossana Lewis

Email: rossanalewis01@gmail.com

TABLE OF CONTENT

Chapter 1: Understanding cystic fibrosis

1.1 Basics of cystic fibrosis

1.2 Genetic Roots

1.3 Diagnosis Simplified

Chapter 2: Empowering Your Health

2.1 Nutrition Essentials

2.2 Exercise for Strength

2.3 Mindfulness Practices

Chapter 3: Medical Insights and Treatments

3.1 Medications and Therapies

3.2 Latest Breakthroughs

3.3 Navigating Medical Procedures

Chapter 4: Daily Management Strategies

4.1 Personalized Care Plans

4.2 Routine Health Monitoring

4.3 Building a Support System

Chapter 5: Coping with Emotional Challenges

5.1 Mental Health Strategies

5.2 Real-life Resilience

5.3 Cultivating a Positive Mindset

Chapter 6: Navigating Relationships

6.1 Family Support Dynamics

6.2 Balancing Relationships

6.3 Advocating for Awareness

Conclusion

Chapter 1: Understanding cystic fibrosis

1.1 Basics of cystic fibrosis

cystic fibrosis is an inherited disease characterized by the buildup of thick, sticky mucus that can damage many of the body's organs. The disorder's most common signs and symptoms include progressive damage to the respiratory system and chronic digestive system problems. The features of the disorder and their severity varies among affected individuals.

Mucus is a slippery substance that lubricates and protects the linings of the airways, digestive system, reproductive system, and other organs and tissues. In people with cystic fibrosis, the body produces mucus that is abnormally thick and sticky. This abnormal mucus can clog the airways leading to severe problems with breathing and bacterial infections in the lungs. These infections cause chronic coughing, wheezing, and inflammation. Over time, mucus buildup and infections result in permanent lung damage, including the formation of scar tissue (fibrosis) and cysts in the lungs.

Most people with cystic fibrosis also have digestive problems. Some affected babies have meconium ileus, a blockage of the intestine that occurs shortly after birth. Other digestive problems result from a buildup of thick, sticky mucus in the pancreas. The pancreas is an organ that produces insulin (a hormone that helps control blood glucose levels). It also makes enzymes that help digest food. In people with cystic fibrosis, mucus often damages the pancreas, impairing its ability to produce insulin and digestive enzymes. Problems with digestion can lead to diarrhea, malnutrition, poor growth, and weight loss. In adolescence or adulthood, a shortage of insulin can cause a form of diabetes known as cystic fibrosis-related diabetes mellitus (CFRDM).

cystic fibrosis used to be considered a fatal disease of childhood. With improved treatments and better ways to manage the disease, many people with cystic fibrosis now live well into adulthood. Adults with cystic fibrosis experience health problems affecting the respiratory, digestive, and reproductive systems. Most men with cystic fibrosis have congenital bilateral absence of the vas deferens (CBAVD), a condition in which the tubes that carry sperm (the vas deferens) are blocked by mucus and do not develop properly. Men with CBAVD are unable to father children (infertile) unless they undergo fertility treatment. Women with cystic fibrosis may experience complications in pregnancy.

1.2 Genetic Roots

Every person inherits two cystic fibrosis Transmembrane Conductance Regulator (CFTR) genes, one gene from each parent. Children who inherit a CFTR gene with a mutation from both parents will have cystic fibrosis. When a mutated CFTR gene is inherited from only one parent and a normal CFTR gene is inherited from the other, the person will be a cystic fibrosis carrier. CF carriers are generally healthy, but they can pass the mutated CFTR gene on to their children. A person inherits two copies of the CFTR gene, one from each parent. If each parent has a normal CFTR gene and a mutated CFTR gene, each child has a 25% chance of inheriting two normal genes, a 50% chance of inheriting one normal gene and one gene with a mutation and being a cystic fibrosis carrier, and a 25% chance of inheriting two genes with mutations and having cystic fibrosis.

Also, at the basic level, we know the genetic cause of cystic fibrosis: it is an autosomal recessive disease caused by mutations in the gene encoding the cystic fibrosis transmembrane conductance regulator (CFTR). At the clinical level, we know that chronic bacterial airway infection, prominent neutrophilic inflammation, mucus-obstructed airways, and progressive bronchiectasis characterize advanced cystic fibrosis lung disease, which causes most cystic fibrosis morbidity and mortality. Between those two extremes, how loss of CFTR-mediated chloride and bicarbonate transport leads to chronic airway infection has remained uncertain.

Over the past two decades, investigators have studied people with cystic fibrosis, who have disease causing CFTR mutations, at progressively earlier time points. We have learned that, by 3 years of age, bronchiectasis is present in nearly one in three children with cystic fibrosis, although the host defense defects that trigger infection continue to be debated. Even before symptom onset, pulmonary inflammation and infection are often present, although which comes first has been uncertain. As early as 3 months of age, most babies with cystic fibrosis have abnormal chest X-ray computed tomography (CT), although the relative contribution of inflammation, airway remodeling or other factors remains undefined. Moving to even earlier time points might reveal the origins of cystic fibrosis lung disease and thereby change clinical practice.

Indeed, simply knowing that disease begins before symptoms has been a factor driving cystic fibrosis centers to intervene early, and the outcomes have been encouraging. Understanding the initial host defense defects in cystic fibrosis airways could suggest novel preventions and treatments and the means to assess disease status and efficacy of therapeutics. Implementation of universal newborn cystic fibrosis screening and potential new therapeutics that target CFTR, further emphasize the need to elucidate the origins of this disease.

1.3 Diagnosis Simplified

Before diving into the diagnosis of cystic fibrosis, let's talk about the symptoms. For classic cystic fibrosis, children who have classic CF have the following symptoms:

- Failure to thrive (inability to gain weight despite having a good appetite and taking in enough calories).
- Loose or oily stools.
- Trouble breathing.
- Recurrent wheezing.
- Frequent lung infections (recurrent pneumonia or bronchitis).
- Recurrent sinus infections.
- A nagging cough.
- Slow growth.

For atypical cystic fibrosis, adults may be mostly diagnosed with it. Respiratory signs and symptoms may include:

- Chronic sinusitis.
- Breathing problems, possibly diagnosed as asthma or chronic obstructive pulmonary disease (COPD).
- Nasal polyps.
- Frequent bouts of pneumonia.

Other signs and symptoms of atypical CF may include:

- Dehydration or heat stroke that reveals abnormal electrolyte levels.
- Fertility problems.
- Diarrhea.
- Pancreatitis.
- Unintended weight loss.

Diagnosis

CF is diagnosed during childhood. Doctors diagnose CF with a thorough evaluation and by using different tests. These include:

Newborn Screening: Your healthcare provider takes a few drops of blood from a heel prick, usually while your newborn is in the hospital, and places the drops on a special card called a Guthrie card. The screening looks for a list of conditions, including CF. Every U.S. state requires the testing of newborns at birth and a few weeks later.

Sweat Test: The sweat test measures the amount of chloride in the body's sweat, which is higher in people who have CF. In the test, your healthcare provider spreads a chemical called pilocarpine on your skin, then applies a small amount of electric stimulation to encourage the sweat glands to produce sweat. Your provider then collects the sweat in a plastic coil or on a piece of filter paper or gauze. People of any age can have a sweat test. It's not painful and does not use a needle. This is the most conclusive test for CF.

Genetic Tests: Blood samples are tested for the gencs that cause CF.

Chest X-rays: Your healthcare provider will order X-rays of the chest used to support or confirm CF, but a chest X-ray isn't the only test needed to confirm a diagnosis. Other tests must be done.

Sinus X-rays: As with chest X-rays, sinus X-rays can confirm CF in people who show certain symptoms. Other forms of testing are used along with sinus X-rays.

Lung Function Tests: The most common lung function test uses a device called a spirometer. You breathe in completely, then push the inhaled breath into the mouthpiece of the spirometer.

Sputum Culture: Your healthcare provider takes a sample of your sputum (spit) and tests it for bacteria. Certain bacteria, such as Pseudomonas, are most commonly found in people who have CF.

Nasal potential difference (NPD): This test uses a voltmeter and electrodes placed in two places in your nose and one place outside of your nose to measure the electricity generated by the transfer of ions in solution across the nasal tissue. The test uses three different types of solutions.

Intestinal Current Measurement (ICM): You'll have to have a biopsy of rectal tissue for this test. The tissue is made to secrete chloride, which is then measured.

In people who have atypical cystic fibrosis, the sweat test may be normal in terms of the levels of chloride. Some people with atypical CF may have been born before testing became routine. Your provider may order NPD and ICM tests when the diagnosis is questionable.

Chapter 2: Empowering Your Health

2.1 Nutrition Essentials

Good nutrition is key for those living with cystic fibrosis (CF). This means: eating a balanced diet, staying hydrated and getting enough calories.

Eating a Balanced Diet

In general, people with CF need 30 to 50 percent more calories daily than others in their age group. Also, 85 to 90 percent of those with CF have pancreatic insufficiency. This happens when the mucus builds up and affects the pancreas. The pancreas is an organ that helps digest food. Your eating plan may include:

Protein: This should make up about 15 to 20 percent of your calories a day. Protein helps build strong muscles. These include meats and fish, eggs, cheese, soy foods and nuts.

Fats: Fatty foods are the richest source of calories. Each gram of fat has nine calories. People with CF should get 35 to 40 percent of their intake from fat. Fat is also a good source of essential fatty acids and fat-soluble vitamins like vitamin A. Choose "good" unsaturated fats when you can. Try olive, corn, soy and sunflower oils. Try these tips to get more fat in your diet:

- Add butter or olive oil to vegetables or over pasta
- Eat chocolate or add whipped cream to puddings and pies
- Always use full fat dressings

Carbohydrates: These are another good source of calories. They can be found in cereals, breads and pastas. Choose pastas made with whole wheat and extra omega-3 fatty acids. Boost your calories by adding dried fruits, whole milk to cereals and nuts.

Calcium: CF puts you at risk for having osteoporosis (weak, brittle bones). Eat more foods with dairy to lower your risk. Look for dairy that's high in fat. Good choices are cream and fruit juices with added calcium.

Essential Fatty Acids: These are often referred to as omega-3 and omega-6 fatty acids, Essential fatty acids are often found in fish oils. They are shown to help develop the brain. They are also good for overall growth. Try salmon and flaxseed oil.

Fat-soluble Vitamins (A, D, E and K): These help promote good eyesight, healthy bones and growth. They help with blood clotting and making red blood cells. CF prevents the body from absorbing these vitamins. You can add these to your diet with a vitamin supplement made just for CF.

Iron: Iron helps to fight infection. It also carries oxygen to cells throughout the body. You can get iron by eating meats, cereals, dried fruits and dark green leafy vegetables.

Zinc: This helps with growth, healing and fighting infection. You can boost zinc in your diet by eating meats, eggs and seafood. Zinc is also found in many multivitamin supplements.

Staying Hydrated

Getting plenty of fluids is good for managing CF. Staying hydrated keeps mucus thinner. It also helps food move along in your gut. With CF, you may not always feel thirsty. That's because CF makes you lose more salt. Know the signs when your body is dehydrated. You may feel tired, dizzy, have headaches or muscle cramps.

Follow these tips to make sure your body gets what it needs:

Eat More Salt: Replace the salt you lose from sweating. This is especially important when you exercise. Add salt to your food, or eat salty snacks like pretzels, salted nuts and chips.

Fill That Bottle: Drink water throughout your day. Try keeping a full water bottle close by. In general, people should drink about 2 liters a day. Younger children may need about 1 to 1.7 liters a day. Talk to your doctor about how much fluid you should drink.

Know Your Drinks: Drink water, milk and sports drinks. Avoid caffeine and alcohol. They can make your body lose fluids instead of hydrating you.

Getting Enough Calories

Many people with CF need to add dietary supplements to their daily diet. This is especially true for children. This helps make sure they get enough calories, protein and nutrients. For example, you can increase your calories by drinking nutritional shakes. You can make these at home or buy them at a store. Many children are picky eaters. Keeping up with calories can be hard if your child also has CF. Try eating meals as a family. Make mealtime a social and fun event. This provides structured time and encourages positive eating habits.

You may also need pancreatic enzymes. They help absorb nutrients from your diet. Your eating plan should fit your needs. Work with your dietitian to find the diet and supplements that work best for you.

2.2 Exercise for Strength

cystic fibrosis (CF) can cause symptoms such as coughing, fatigue, and difficulty breathing, which may make it challenging to exercise. However, regular exercise can help improve lung function, increase strength, and boost endurance, increasing your overall physical fitness. Exercising can also positively affect mental health by reducing anxiety and depression. Whether you're just starting or looking to take your fitness to the next level, this guide can help you develop an exercise routine that fits your goals and abilities. It's important to start slowly and gradually increase the intensity and duration of the exercise over time. This helps ensure you can sustain your routine while preventing injury and overexertion.

Before starting an exercise program, consult with a healthcare professional to determine the appropriate type and intensity of exercise for your needs.

Aerobic Exercises

There are aerobic exercises a patient can try also known as cardio. They help increase your heart rate, improve circulation, and enhance respiratory function. These activities can be an enjoyable way to incorporate physical activity into your daily life. Start with 5-minute sessions and gradually build up the duration and intensity as you progress. Cardio exercises that may be beneficial for people living with CF include: swimming, walking, jogging, cycling, rowing, hiking, dancing.

Resistance Training Exercises

Plank: This bodyweight exercise targets your shoulders, core, and hamstrings. It also helps develop balance, stability, and strength, which can improve posture.

To do this:

- Start on all fours, with your hands shoulder-width apart.

- Extend your legs, lift your heels, and raise your hips to align your spine.

- Engage your abdominal, arm, and leg muscles to stabilize your body.

- Extend the back of your neck, relax your throat, and gaze toward the floor.

- Hold this position for up to 1 minute.

Resistance Band Rows: For this exercise, you need a resistance band. This move targets the rhomboid and trapezius muscles, helping to increase scapular stability and upper body strength.

To do this:

- Anchor a resistance band to a stable object, such as a door or pole.

- Stand with your feet hip-width apart.

- Hold the resistance band with both hands at or slightly below chest level.
- Pull the band toward your body, drawing your shoulder blades together.
- Maintain proper posture and alignment.
- Do 2–4 sets of 8–12 repetitions.

Stretches

Thoracic Extension: This stretch helps improve posture, promotes spinal mobility, and enhances overall flexibility. It may be especially beneficial if you spend long periods sitting or standing.

To do this:
- Sit on a chair or cushion.
- Interlace your fingers behind your head.
- Gently arch your upper back while squeezing your shoulder blades together.

- Create resistance by pressing your hands into your head.
- Hold this position for up to 30 seconds.

Cat Cow: This yoga posture helps increase spinal flexibility and alleviates neck, shoulder, and back tension.

To do this:

- Start in a tabletop position with your wrists under your shoulders and your knees under your hips.
- Inhale and arch your back, lowering your stomach toward the floor.
- Lift your head and tailbone toward the ceiling.

- Exhale and round your spine, tucking your chin toward your chest and drawing your navel toward your spine.
- Move slowly, continuing this fluid movement.
- Continue for up to 1 minute.

Quadriceps Stretch: This stretch targets the front of your thigh to alleviate tension and soreness. It also increases flexibility in your hips and knees.

To do this:

- Stand next to a wall or a chair for balance.
- Bend your right knee and bring your heel toward your buttocks.
- Hold onto your ankle or foot with your right hand.

- Extend your left arm out to the side or straight overhead.

- Keep your knees together in the same plane and maintain proper posture.

- Hold for up to 30 seconds.

- Repeat on the opposite side.

Breathing Exercises

Breathing exercises increase lung capacity, develop breath awareness, and promote relaxation. You can do them throughout the day and during activities that cause shortness of breath.

Pursed Lip Breathing: This breathing exercise encourages relaxation, reduces shortness of breath, and helps release air trapped in the lungs.

To do this:

- Sit comfortably and relax your shoulders.
- Inhale slowly through your nose for 2–3 seconds.
- Purse your lips and exhale slowly for 4–6 seconds.
- Continue for a few minutes.

Huff Coughing: This breathing technique helps clear mucus from your airways.

To do this:

- Take a deep breath.
- Exhale forcefully while making a "ha" sound.
- Repeat several times to move the mucus up to your larger airways.

- Continue until you huff all of the mucus out of your lungs.

Diaphragmatic Breathing: This breathing exercise has a calming effect, helps to expand your lungs, and improves airflow. You can do it a few times throughout the day. Pay attention to the sensation of your breath and the movement of your hands as you breathe, and use the following steps:

- Lie on your back with a pillow under your knees.
- To alleviate low back pain, bend your knees with your feet flat on the floor.
- Place one hand on your chest and the other on your stomach.
- Inhale deeply through your nose, allowing your stomach to expand with air.

- Exhale slowly through pursed lips, drawing your abdomen in toward your spine.
- Continue for up to 5 minutes.

2.3 Mindfulness Practices

Through meditation practices, mindfulness encourages a focus on how you're feeling in the moment, clearing your mind of any judgments and thoughts about the future. It uses different breathing and thinking techniques to make you feel more relaxed and grounded.

Mindfulness can help people with respiratory conditions like pulmonary fibrosis by restoring control when they are anxious or out of breath. It is easy to get the hang of. You can practice mindfulness anywhere as long as you have the ability to feel calm and comfortable – although a quiet place is best. It can help people with health conditions that are caused or worsened by anxiety and stress.

How mindfulness works

If you're new to mindfulness, try this simple breathing exercise and consider the following:

- Take note of how much your breathing starts to slow, and how relaxed you become as a result

- Notice if your mind starts to wander; when it does, try to focus back on your breath, the noises in your surroundings and the space around you

- Do not be hard on yourself if you struggle to relax or clear your mind. Remember that some days you will find it easier than others

- Shift focus away from your lungs if you are anxious and out of breath. Instead, gently move your attention to your nostrils, focusing on how the air feels cold as it goes in through your nose, and warm as it comes out through your mouth

Practicing these mindfulness techniques regularly can:

- Help you deal with stress and anxiety in the moment when they happen
- Support you to avoid re-activating your 'fight or flight' alarm system in the future

Chapter 3: Medical Insights and Treatments

3.1 Medications and Therapies

While there is not yet a cure for cystic fibrosis, advances in treatment are helping people live longer, healthier lives. To better manage your condition, you or your child will work with cystic fibrosis specialists. In newborns with a positive screening result, treatment may begin while the diagnosis is being confirmed. Treatment for cystic fibrosis is focused on airway clearance, medicines to improve the function of the faulty CFTR protein and prevent complications, and surgery, if needed.

Medicines to treat cystic fibrosis include those used to maintain and improve lung function, fight infections, clear mucus and help breathing, and work on the faulty CFTR protein.

Antibiotics: Prevent or treat lung infections and improve lung function. Your doctor may prescribe oral, inhaled, or intravenous (IV) antibiotics.

Anti-inflammatory Medicines: such as ibuprofen or corticosteroids, reduce inflammation. Inflammation causes many of the changes in cystic fibrosis, such as lung disease. Ibuprofen is especially beneficial for children, but side effects can include kidney and stomach problems. Corticosteroids can cause bone thinning and increased blood sugar and blood pressure.

Bronchodilators: relax and open airways. These treatments are taken by inhaling them.

CFTR Modulators: improve the function of the faulty CFTR protein. They improve lung function and help prevent lung problems and other complications. Examples include ivacaftor and lumacaftor and a triple combination medicine (elexacaftor–tezacaftor–ivacaftor). The combination medicine is the first approved treatment that may help up to 90% of people who have cystic fibrosis. It is currently approved to use in adults and children older than 12 years.

Mucus Thinners: make it easier to clear the mucus from your airways. These treatments are taken by inhaling them.

There are many different procedures a cystic fibrosis patient need to undergo

Airway Clearance Techniques: Airway clearance techniques also called chest physical therapy (CPT) can relieve mucus obstruction and help to reduce infection and inflammation in the airways. These techniques loosen the thick mucus in the lungs, making it easier to cough up. Airway clearing techniques are usually done several times a day. Different types of CPT can be used to loosen and remove mucus, and a combination of techniques may be recommended.

- A common technique is clapping with cupped hands on the front and back of the chest.

- Certain breathing and coughing techniques also may be used to help loosen the mucus.

- Mechanical devices can help loosen lung mucus. Devices include a tube that you blow into and a machine that pulses air into the lungs (vibrating vest). Vigorous exercise also may be used to clear mucus.

Your doctor will instruct you on the type and frequency of chest physical therapy that's best for you.

Pulmonary Rehabilitation: Your doctor may recommend a long-term program that may improve your lung function and overall well-being. Pulmonary rehabilitation is usually done on an outpatient basis and may include:

- Physical exercise that may improve your condition
- Breathing techniques that may help loosen mucus and improve breathing
- Nutritional counseling
- Counseling and support

- Education about your condition

Options for certain conditions caused by cystic fibrosis include:

Nasal and Sinus Surgery: Your doctor may recommend surgery to remove nasal polyps that obstruct breathing. Sinus surgery may be done to treat recurrent or chronic sinusitis.

Oxygen Therapy: If your blood oxygen level declines, your doctor may recommend that you breathe pure oxygen to prevent high blood pressure in the lungs (pulmonary hypertension).

Noninvasive Ventilation: Typically used while sleeping, noninvasive ventilation uses a nose or mouth mask to provide positive pressure in the airway and lungs when you breathe in. It's often used in combination with oxygen therapy.

Noninvasive ventilation can increase air exchange in the lungs and decrease the work of breathing. The treatment may also help with airway clearance.

Feeding Tube: cystic fibrosis interferes with digestion, so you can't absorb nutrients from food very well. Your doctor may suggest using a feeding tube to deliver extra nutrition. This tube may be a temporary tube inserted into your nose and guided to your stomach, or the tube may be surgically implanted in the abdomen. The tube can be used to give extra calories during the day or night and does not prevent eating by mouth.

Bowel Surgery: If a blockage develops in your bowel, you may need surgery to remove it. Intussusception, where a segment of intestine has telescoped inside an adjacent section of intestine, also may require surgical repair.

Lung Transplant: If you have severe breathing problems, life-threatening lung complications or increasing resistance to antibiotics for lung infections, lung transplantation may be an option. Because bacteria line the airways in diseases that cause permanent widening of the large airways (bronchiectasis), such as cystic fibrosis, both lungs need to be replaced. cystic fibrosis does not recur in transplanted lungs. However, other complications associated with CF such as sinus infections, diabetes, pancreas conditions and osteoporosis can still occur after a lung transplant.

Liver Transplant: For severe cystic fibrosis-related liver disease, such as cirrhosis, liver transplant may be an option. In some people, a liver transplant may be combined with lung or pancreas transplants.

3.2 Latest Breakthroughs

In October 2019, the U.S Food and Drug Association (FDA) authorized a new era in cystic fibrosis (CF) treatment. For the first time, the FDA has approved an oral medication that targets a gene defect responsible for approximately 90% of the 80,000 CF cases worldwide. The new drug, TRIKAFTA, was approved after a series of landmark clinical trials – including research conducted at the UT Southwestern cystic fibrosis Clinic – in which patients with one or more Phe508del gene mutations experienced dramatic positive outcomes. The findings were published and showed that when compared with placebo, the drug: significantly improved lung function at four weeks, which was sustained through 24 weeks, reduced lung flare-ups by 63%, decreased the amount of salt lost through sweating, improved patients' short-term quality of life and respiratory symptom scores.

In some cases, the drug has been so effective that patients have been removed from the lung transplant list. However, TRIKAFTA is not curative and not all patients will experience similar results. While generally considered safe, long-term research is needed to understand potential side effects of the drug over years of treatment.

TRIKAFTA is an oral drug, which is a major shift from the time-consuming nebulizer therapies people with CF are accustomed to. It is currently approved for people 12 and older with one or more Phe508del gene mutations. For these people, the drug has potential to turn a once fatal disease into a more manageable condition – and hope for more effective therapies for patients with other mutations.

3.3 Navigating Medical Procedures

First, one needs to understand the condition of cystic fibrosis. As it is a genetic disorder that affects the lungs, pancreas, and other organs. Second, understand the treatment options. Treatment for cystic fibrosis has changed significantly in recent years, with many new and improved therapies becoming available. The first step in navigating treatment options is to work with a multidisciplinary team of healthcare providers, including a pulmonologist, a respiratory therapist, a dietician, and a social worker. This team can help to develop a personalized treatment plan, which may include:

- Medications such as bronchodilators, anti-inflammatories, and antibiotics.
- Airway clearance therapy, such as chest physiotherapy and the use of devices to loosen and clear mucus.

Third, understand the importance of lifestyle management. In addition to medical procedures, a treatment plan for cystic fibrosis should also include lifestyle management strategies. These can include:

- Nutrition and dietary management, to make sure the body is getting enough calories and nutrients to support the lungs.
- Exercise, to improve lung function and overall well-being.

- Stress management, to reduce the impact of stress on the body.

- Emotional support, to help cope with the challenges of living with cystic fibrosis.

- Vaccinations, to prevent infections that can be especially dangerous for individuals with cystic fibrosis.

Chapter 4: Daily Management Strategies

4.1 Personalized Care Plans

Personalized care plans, in the context of healthcare, are tailored and individualized strategies designed to address the specific needs, preferences, and conditions of an individual. These plans take into account various aspects of a person's health, lifestyle, and medical history to provide targeted and effective interventions. In the case of cystic fibrosis, personalized care plans are comprehensive strategies that go beyond a one-size-fits-all approach. They consider the unique combination of symptoms, genetic factors, and lifestyle considerations that characterize each individual's experience with cystic fibrosis.

Key components of personalized care plans for cystic fibrosis typically include:

Comprehensive Health Assessment: An initial evaluation that involves a thorough examination of respiratory function, nutritional status, and psychosocial well-being. This assessment establishes a baseline of the individual's health and informs the development of the care plan.

Nutritional Considerations: Tailored dietary plans that address the specific nutritional needs of individuals with cystic fibrosis. This may include adjustments in calorie intake, specialized diets, and the integration of enzyme replacement therapies.

Respiratory and Physical Therapies: Customized approaches to respiratory care, including personalized airway clearance techniques, inhalation therapies, and exercise regimens designed to optimize lung function and physical well-being.

Psychosocial Support: Provisions for emotional and mental well-being, recognizing the psychosocial impact of cystic fibrosis. This may involve access to counseling services, participation in support groups, and strategies for coping with the emotional aspects of living with a chronic condition.

Collaborative Approach: Active collaboration between the individual, their family, and the healthcare team. This ensures that the care plan aligns with the individual's preferences, values, and goals. The plan is designed to be flexible, allowing for adjustments based on the individual's evolving health needs.

Overall, personalized care plans aim to optimize the overall quality of life for individuals with cystic fibrosis by tailoring interventions to their unique health profile. These plans are dynamic and may evolve over time based on ongoing assessments and the individual's response to interventions.

4.2 Routine Health Monitoring

Routine health monitoring is a crucial component of personalized care plans for individuals with cystic fibrosis. This ongoing process involves regular assessments, tests, and check-ups to track the individual's health status, adjust interventions as needed, and proactively manage the impact of cystic fibrosis on various aspects of well-being.

Frequency of Monitoring: Establish a schedule for routine health monitoring that aligns with the individual's unique needs. This may involve regular check-ups with healthcare providers, periodic assessments of respiratory function, and nutritional evaluations.

Lung Function Tests: Incorporate regular lung function tests into the monitoring routine. Spirometry and other pulmonary function tests assess the efficiency of the respiratory system. Changes in lung function can indicate the progression of cystic fibrosis and guide adjustments to treatment plans.

Nutritional Assessments: Integrate nutritional assessments into routine monitoring to track the individual's nutritional status. Measurements of weight, height, and body mass index (BMI) provide valuable insights into the effectiveness of dietary interventions and the overall impact on growth and well-being.

Psychosocial Evaluations: Include psychosocial evaluations as part of routine monitoring. Assessing mental and emotional well-being allows healthcare providers to identify and address any challenges related to the psychosocial impact of living with cystic fibrosis.

Medication Reviews: Regularly review and adjust medications as needed. Routine monitoring includes assessing the effectiveness of prescribed medications, managing potential side effects, and ensuring optimal adherence to the treatment plan.

Collaborative Discussions: Engage in collaborative discussions during routine health monitoring sessions. Actively involve the individual with cystic fibrosis, their family, and the healthcare team in open communication. Discuss any changes in symptoms, challenges, or preferences to inform adjustments to the care plan.

Imaging Studies: Consider periodic imaging studies, such as chest X-rays or CT scans, as part of routine health monitoring. These studies provide detailed insights into the condition of the lungs and assist in identifying any structural changes or complications.

Laboratory Tests: Conduct routine laboratory tests to assess various health markers, including blood counts and liver function. Monitoring these parameters helps healthcare providers identify potential complications early on and adjust interventions accordingly.

Educational Updates: Use routine health monitoring sessions as opportunities for educational updates. Provide information on the latest advancements in cystic fibrosis management, self-care practices, and any changes in treatment approaches.

Documentation and Tracking: Maintain comprehensive documentation of routine health monitoring results. Create a record that tracks changes over time, helping healthcare providers and individuals alike visualize progress and make informed decisions about the ongoing care plan.

4.3 Building a Support System

Living with CF, we become experts in our care. We must learn to manage the physical, psychological, and social challenges of living each day with a chronic disease. Building a support system is necessary to help you cope. They provide encouragement and support your needs when things are difficult and also create accountability to help avoid cutting corners when things are going well.

Here are tips you may need to build a support system:
Allow Friends and Family to Help, Even with the Small Stuff: Don't let pride get in your way.

Even if you think you can do it yourself, allowing others to do even small things to help gives them a sense of purpose and importance and shows that you love and trust them.

Exercise is a Great Source of "Bonding": Going for a walk, run, or bike ride, or to an exercise class can be a great opportunity to bond with people you care about. In addition to the health benefits, it's a great time to talk and share. It also often provides a great opportunity for them to ask questions about how you're doing and for you to open up about how you're feeling.

Let Others See You Do Your Treatments: Especially a roommate, boyfriend, or girlfriend. It's easy to keep many aspects of CF hidden. Sharing the realities of your treatment routine will help others understand what you contend with day in and day out. Take pride in the amount of work you do to stay healthy. In my experience, helping others to understand what you need to do to help maintain your regimen creates respect, not pity.

Accept CF as Part of Your Life: Exercise, eating well, following doctor's orders, and having fun are all contributing factors to a good life, with or without CF. So, too, are friends and family! The more open you can be with your friends and family about how CF is affecting you, the more support they can provide in both good times and bad.

Surround Yourself With People Who Inspire You: Be selective about those you choose to spend your time with. Build relationships with people you admire and who motivate and support you. There will be those you come across who may feel pity for you or choose to leave you out. Remember, your time and energy are valuable. Only share yourself with those who deserve it.

Choose to invest in building relationships that make your life better and happier. There are aspects of your life that are not fun, so creating a support system of family, friends and healthcare providers that you trust and can talk openly with will be critically important for you as you manage cystic fibrosis.

Chapter 5: Coping With Emotional Challenges

5.1 Mental Health Strategies

Research has shown that people with chronic diseases (defined as a condition that persists for longer than three months) can often have anxiety and depression. It is estimated that up to one third of individuals with a serious medical condition will experience depression. Depression is one of the most common complications of chronic illnesses like cystic fibrosis.

As an individual with CF, it's important to be aware of this and ensure that you identify and communicate these feelings so that you can receive support.

Adolescents and adults may experience occasional periods of feeling down. For some individuals with a good support network, these feelings can improve. For others, symptoms may occur over prolonged periods of time and feelings of self-doubt and sadness may become overwhelming.

Depression is identified by a variety of symptoms. If you have five or more of the following symptoms present over a two week period, it's important that you consult your health care provider. He/she will ask you questions about your wellbeing and overall mood.

- Sadness/irritability
- Changes in weight/appetite
- Guilt, hopelessness or worthlessness

- Inability to concentrate, remembering things or making decisions
- Fatigue/loss of energy
- Loss of interest in sex and other activities once enjoyed
- Sleep disturbances
- Restlessness or decreased activity
- Physical aches and pains with no medical cause
- Thoughts of suicide or death

Another common mental health concern that may, or may not, accompany depression is anxiety. Anxiety is a feeling of worry that may include nervousness or agitation. Everyone may experience this on a short term basis, but prolonged feelings of anxiety, may lead to cognitive, physical and behavioural symptoms.

One of the most common forms of anxiety is Generalized Anxiety Disorder (GAD). GAD is defined as excessive anxiety and worry i.e. apprehensive expectation, occurring more days than not for at least six months. It could relate to, a number of events or activities such as work or school performance. The individual is unable to control the worry and the anxiety, GAD is associated with at least three of the following six symptoms:

- Restlessness or feeling 'keyed up' or on edge
- Being easily fatigued
- Difficulty concentrating or mind going blank
- Irritability
- Muscle tension

- Sleep disturbance such as difficulty falling or staying asleep, or restless, unsatisfying sleep.

The anxiety, worry, or physical symptoms cause clinically significant distress or impairment in social, occupational or other important areas of functioning. Similar to depression, it is important to consult your health care practitioner if you feel you are developing symptoms of GAD. Prolonged worry or anxiety can affect your ability to complete tasks. Appropriate help can ensure you have the tools to assist with day to day stress.

5.2 Real-life Resilience

One aspect of resilience that's important for people with cystic fibrosis is self-care. This can involve a range of things, from getting enough sleep and eating a healthy diet to finding ways to relax and de-stress. Self-care is important because it helps people to manage their physical and emotional health, which in turn helps them to cope with the challenges of living with cystic fibrosis.

Another aspect of resilience is finding purpose and meaning in life. This can be achieved through a variety of ways, such as pursuing hobbies and interests, being involved in a community, and making a difference in the world. For example, some people with cystic fibrosis have found purpose by advocating for better treatment options, raising awareness about the disease, and helping others who are going through similar experiences. It's often said that helping others is one of the best ways to help yourself, and this is certainly true for people with cystic fibrosis.

Also, another aspect of resilience for people with cystic fibrosis is finding a support network. This can include friends and family, as well as other people with cystic fibrosis. A support network can provide emotional and practical support, and it can also be a source of information and advice. Many people with cystic fibrosis find strength in knowing that they're not alone and that others understand what they're going through. Support networks can be found both in person and online, and they can be a lifeline for people living with cystic fibrosis.

Furthermore, you also need to embrace its limitations. This doesn't mean giving up on life or giving in to disease, rather, finding ways to live a fulfilling life within the constraints of the disease. For example, some people with this ailment have found new passions and ways to enjoy life despite the limitations of the disease.

5.3 Cultivating a Positive Mindset

This is about more than just "thinking positive" - it's about making an active effort to focus on the good things in life and to look for opportunities for growth. It's not always easy, but it can be very effective in building resilience. Some people with cystic fibrosis have found that gratitude practices, such as writing down things they're grateful for, can be a powerful tool for cultivating a positive mindset. Now let's talk about the power of perspective. This is about recognizing that even in difficult circumstances, there are always two sides to the story. In the case of cystic fibrosis, this can mean recognizing that even though the disease brings many challenges, it can also bring opportunities for growth and new experiences. For example, many people with cystic fibrosis have found new meaning in their lives by connecting with others, sharing their story, and making a difference in the world.

Focus on the present moment, this means being mindful of the here and now rather than dwelling on the past or worrying about the future and also practice mindfulness like we earlier discussed.

Chapter 6: Navigating Relationships

6.1 Family Support Dynamics

When it comes to family support dynamics, there are a few things to keep in mind. First, it's important for families to be supportive of the individual with cystic fibrosis, while also being aware of the challenges that come with the condition. This includes providing emotional support, as well as helping with the practical aspects of living with cystic fibrosis, such as assisting with treatments and medication. In addition, it's important for families to find ways to maintain their own health and well-being, as the stress of caring for a loved one with cystic fibrosis can take a toll. Another important factor is the importance of creating a sense of normalcy. It's crucial for families to find ways to balance the medical needs of the individual with cystic fibrosis with the need for the family to have a normal, happy life. This could include finding ways to have fun together, celebrating achievements, and making sure that everyone has time to pursue their own interests and hobbies. It's also important for families to find ways to support each other and not feel isolated or alone.

In healthy families, there is open and honest communication, support for the individual with cystic fibrosis, and balance between the needs of everyone in the family. In unhealthy families, the needs of the individual with cystic fibrosis can take precedence over everything else, leading to resentment and burnout. Additionally, families who do not prioritize self-care can find themselves overwhelmed and unable to provide effective support.

6.2 Balancing Relationships

First, it's important to understand the demands that cystic fibrosis places on an individual. For example, they may have frequent doctor's appointments, time-consuming treatments, and medication regimens that take up a lot of their time. In addition, they may experience feelings of isolation and loneliness due to the limitations that cystic fibrosis places on their social life. It's important to recognize these demands and to communicate them to loved ones. Now, how can we balance relationships and also meet the demands of cystic fibrosis? One way is to set boundaries with loved ones. For example, individuals with cystic fibrosis may need to set limits on the amount of time they can spend socializing or may need to cancel plans at the last minute due to illness. By setting these boundaries, they can avoid feelings of guilt or resentment from both themselves and their loved ones. Additionally, individuals can find creative ways to spend time with loved ones that don't place too much strain on their health. Another important factor in balancing relationships is finding the right support system. It's important to surround oneself with individuals who are understanding and supportive of the demands of cystic fibrosis. This might include family members, friends, or members of a cystic fibrosis support group. By finding the right support system, individuals can feel understood and cared for, which can help them to maintain their relationships. In addition, support systems can also provide practical assistance, such as helping with household chores or providing transportation to appointments.

In addition to finding the right support system, individuals with cystic fibrosis can also benefit from finding ways to connect with others who have the same condition. Connecting with others who have cystic fibrosis can provide a sense of belonging and understanding that can be difficult to find elsewhere. It can also provide an opportunity to share tips and strategies for managing the disease. There are many ways to connect with others with cystic fibrosis, such as joining online forums, attending support groups, or attending a camp for individuals with cystic fibrosis.

Finally, it's important to make time for self-care when balancing relationships and cystic fibrosis.

Self-care can take many forms, such as taking breaks from socializing, engaging in hobbies, and getting enough sleep. By making time for self-care, individuals can recharge their energy and prevent burnout. This, in turn, can help them to have more to give in their relationships. Self-care is an important part of maintaining balance and preventing the negative effects of stress.

6.3 Advocating for Awareness

Advocacy for awareness is a powerful tool in fostering understanding, driving research, and creating a supportive community. This section focuses on the importance of advocacy and awareness-raising efforts in relation to cystic fibrosis. It explores how raising awareness of cystic fibrosis in different contexts, such as the media, the healthcare system, and the legal system, can have a significant impact on individuals with the condition. By increasing understanding and knowledge about cystic fibrosis, advocacy efforts can lead to improved quality of life for those affected by the disease.

Educational Campaigns: Advocacy involves organizing educational campaigns to disseminate accurate information about cystic fibrosis. Real-life advocacy efforts focus on schools, workplaces, and public forums to increase awareness and dispel misconceptions.

Community Engagement: Engaging the broader community is crucial in advocacy. Real-life initiatives may include organizing events, walks, or fundraisers to raise funds for research, support programs, and create a platform for affected individuals and families to share their stories.

Legislative Advocacy: Advocacy extends to influencing policies and legislations that benefit individuals with cystic fibrosis. Real-life advocacy may involve lobbying for improved healthcare access, increased funding for research, or policies supporting better treatment options.

Social Media Activism: Harnessing the power of social media platforms plays a pivotal role in advocacy. Real-life advocacy involves creating awareness campaigns, sharing personal stories, and fostering online communities for support and information exchange.

Media Outreach: Collaborating with media outlets can significantly amplify advocacy efforts. Real-life stories shared through documentaries, interviews, or articles raise awareness, depict real experiences, and garner public attention towards cystic fibrosis.

Partnerships and Collaborations: Effective advocacy often involves partnerships with organizations, healthcare providers, and influencers. Real-life collaborations may lead to impactful awareness initiatives, resource sharing, and a unified voice advocating for the needs of those with cystic fibrosis.

Educating Healthcare Professionals: Advocacy extends to educating healthcare professionals about the latest advancements and needs of individuals with cystic fibrosis. Real-life initiatives involve workshops, seminars, or publications aimed at enhancing healthcare delivery and understanding of the condition.

Empowering Individuals: Advocacy empowers individuals affected by cystic fibrosis to become advocates themselves. Real-life initiatives focus on providing tools, platforms, and training to enable individuals to share their stories, advocate for their needs, and inspire others.

Global Awareness Efforts: Advocacy transcends borders, aiming for global awareness and support. Real-life efforts may involve collaborations with international organizations, fostering a global network for information exchange and support.

Conclusion

In the journey through the complexities of cystic fibrosis, each chapter, story, and experience intricately weaves a tapestry of resilience, strength, and unwavering determination. As we draw this comprehensive guide to a close, the resounding message echoes loud and clear: hope thrives, and resilience knows no bounds.

This exploration into the multifaceted world of cystic fibrosis has been a testament to the unwavering spirit of individuals, families, and communities. From understanding the genetic roots to navigating the intricacies of diagnosis and treatment, from fostering resilient relationships to advocating for awareness, every facet unveils the unwavering resolve of those touched by this condition.

In the face of challenges, families have emerged as pillars of support, fostering understanding and navigating the delicate balance between caregiving and fostering independence. Individuals with cystic fibrosis have showcased immeasurable strength, embracing life's milestones, advocating for themselves, and inspiring others with their resilience.

As we conclude this journey, it's imperative to recognize that the pursuit of advancements, both in medical research and societal support, remains pivotal. Every voice raised in advocacy, every step taken in raising awareness, and every effort made in fostering understanding contributes to a future brimming with possibilities.

The journey doesn't end here; it continues, fueled by hope, resilience, and the collective efforts of a community dedicated to triumphing over challenges. Each story shared, each lesson learned, and each act of advocacy propels us forward, nurturing hope and forging a path towards a world where cystic fibrosis does not define limits, but rather inspires resilience.

May this guide serve as a beacon of empowerment, an ode to the unwavering strength within each individual, and a catalyst for continued advocacy and progress in the realm of cystic fibrosis. Together, we stand united in the pursuit of a future where every step forward is a testament to triumph over adversity.

If you're reading this book on cystic fibrosis, you may also be interested in my book on osteoporosis and lung cancer. Tap the links above to read them.

www.ingramcontent.com/pod-product-compliance
Lightning Source LLC
Chambersburg PA
CBHW050834260726
48660CB00006B/2233